Copycat Japanese Recipes for Beginners

A Step-by-Step Guide to Making the Most Popular and Favorite Japanese Restaurant Dishes for Beginners.

By Sakura Tanaka

© **Copyright 2021 - All rights reserved.**

The content contained within this book may not be reproduced, duplicated or transmitted without direct written permission from the author or the publisher.

Under no circumstances will any blame or legal responsibility be held against the publisher, or author, for any damages, reparation, or monetary loss due to the information contained within this book. Either directly or indirectly.

Legal Notice:

This book is copyright protected. This book is only for personal use. You cannot amend, distribute, sell, use, quote or paraphrase any part, or the content within this book, without the consent of the author or publisher.

Disclaimer Notice:

Please note the information contained within this document is for educational and entertainment purposes only. All effort has been executed to present accurate, up to date, and reliable, complete information. No warranties of any kind are declared or implied. Readers acknowledge that the author is not engaging in the rendering of legal, financial, medical or professional advice. The content within this book has been derived from various sources. Please consult a licensed professional before attempting any techniques outlined in this book.

By reading this document, the reader agrees that under no circumstances is the author responsible for any losses, direct or indirect, which are incurred as a result of the use of information contained within this document, including, but not limited to, — errors, omissions, or inaccuracies.

Sommario

Introduction 5

Chapter 1: Rice Recipes 7
    Spam Onigirazu 7
    Seikhan 10
    TamagoKakeGohan 12
    KuriGohan 14
    MameGohan 16
    Matsutake Gohan 18
    Mini Okonomiyaki 20

Chapter 2: Vegetable Recipes 23
    Kabocha Gratin 23
    Daigaku Imo 28
    Carrot Ginger Dressing 31
    Edamame Shichimi 33
    Hijiki No Nimono 35
    Okra Ohitashi 38
    Japanese Pickled Cabbage 40

Chapter 3: Poultry Recipes 42
    Chicken Teriyaki 42
    Teba Shio 45
    Oyakodon 48
    Tsukune 51
    Soboro Don 54

Chapter 4: Seafood Recipes 57
    Unagi Chazuke 57
    Kaki Fry 60
    Smoked Ocean Trout and Noodles 62
    Miso Butter Snapper 64
    KinmedaiNitsuke 67

Chapter 5: Udon and Soba Noodles Recipes 69
    Curry Udon Noodles 69

    Kitsune Udon 71
    Momofuku Soy Sauce Eggs, Chili Chicken, and Soba Noodles
    74
    Soba Noodle and Broccolini Salad 77
    Soba, Prawn, and Lemongrass Soup 79

Chapter 6: Tofu Recipes 83
    Goya Champuru 83
    Hiyayakko 86
    Tofu Pizza 88

Chapter 7: Sushi Recipes 91
    Dragon Rolls 91
    California Rolls 94
    Cucumber Wrapped Sushi 96
    Saba Oshizushi 98

Chapter 8: Soup Recipes 101
    Tonjiru 101
    Matsutake Clear Soup 105
    Tofu and Japanese Pumpkin soup 108
    Champon 110

Chapter 9: Snacks & Dessert Recipes 115
    Mochi Ice Cream 115
    Anmitsu 118
    Fruit Jelly 120
    Warabi Mochi 123
    Yatsuhashi 126

Conclusion 128

Introduction

Hello everyone, do you love the East and all its fascinating world?

Do you love sushi and fish?

Then you have bought the right book!

I will introduce you to a boundless variety of different gastronomical delights that are authentic to Japan, and in the first chapter, you will also learn about what makes Japanese cuisine so unique. Each area of Japan has its own specialty in terms of cuisine, but here, you are going to get a comprehensive approach to all these dishes.

There are plenty of books on this subject on the market, thanks again for choosing this one! Every effort was made to ensure it is full of as much useful information as possible, and please enjoy it!

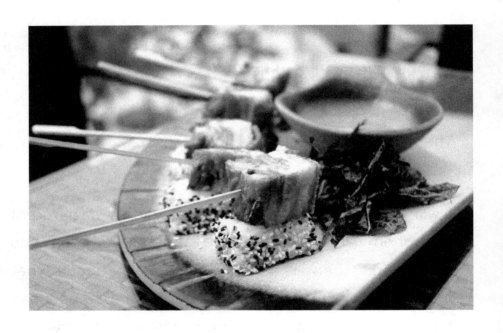

Chapter 1: Rice Recipes

Spam Onigirazu

Total Prep & Cooking Time: 30 minutes

Yields: 6 servings

Nutrition Facts: Calories: 266 | Carbs: 35g | Protein: 11g | Fat: 6g | Fiber: 0g

Ingredients:

- One SPAM product
- Six eggs (large-sized)
- Six lettuce leaves
- Six sheets of nori
- One tbsp. of canola oil
- One tbsp. of furikake
- Three cups of Japanese rice (cooked)
- Kosher salt

For the seasonings:

- One tbsp. each of
- Soy sauce
- Sake
- Mirin

Method:

1. Heat oil in a frying pan and cook the eggs the way you prefer them. Once done, transfer to a plate.

2. Cut the spam into quarter-inch pieces. Add these slices to the pan and cook them until both sides have adequately become browned. Take them out on a plate once they are done.

3. Now, turn down the flame and add the seasonings. Mix well. Add the spam slices into the pan again.

4. On your working surface, keep a plastic wrap, and on top of it, place a sheet of nori seaweed. Spread rice thinly and make sure it has a square shape. Sprinkle

furikake and kosher salt on top. Then, add the fried egg followed by the spam.

5. After that, place a leaf of lettuce and, finally, cover with another thin layer of rice. If you have been using anonigirazu mold for the process, press down the lid slightly and take it back up. Fold the sheets and cover it properly. Use a knife to cut through the center and serve.

Seikhan

Total Prep & Cooking Time: 9 hours 5 minutes

Yields: 5 servings

Nutrition Facts: Calories: 284 | Carbs: 128g | Protein: 14g | Fat: 2g | Fiber: 7g

Ingredients:

- Half a cup each of
- Uncooked Japanese rice
- Azuki beans
- Half a tsp. of kosher salt
- 2.5 cups of water
- Three cups of Mochigome or sweet rice
- Optional – toasted sesame seeds

Method:

1. Soak the azuki beans (for about half a day) after washing them thoroughly.

2. Take a bowl and combine the Japanese rice and Mochigome together and wash them. Drain them.

3. In a small-sized pot, add the azuki beans and then pour just as much water as is needed to cover the beans. Boil the beans. Once they start boiling, turn off the flame and drain them.

4. Place the beans in the same pot again and add 2.5 cups of water. Boil them. Cover the lid and allow them to simmer for fifteen minutes. Reserve the water and beans in separate bowls. The bowl containing the beans will have to be covered by a plastic wrap, and then you have to allow them to cool down.

5. In a rice cooker, add the rice and also add the reserved water from the beans. Then, season with salt and add the beans too. Once they have been cooked, allow them to rest for fifteen minutes with the lid closed. Sprinkle some toasted sesame seeds before serving.

TamagoKakeGohan

Total Prep & Cooking Time: 5 minutes

Yields: 1 serving

Nutrition Facts: Calories: 282 | Carbs: 46g | Protein: 11g | Fat: 5g | Fiber: 1g

Ingredients:

- One egg (keep another egg for optional egg yolk)
- One cup of Japanese rice (cooked)
- Kosher salt
- Soy sauce
- Mirin
- MSG powder
- Torn nori
- Furikake
- Hondashi

Method:

1. First, add the rice to a bowl of your choice and make a hole or indentation right at the center.

2. Take the egg and break it at the center. Add the seasonings. Stir properly so that the egg is well incorporated and becomes fluffy.

3. Sprinkle nori and furikake on top and serve. You can add another egg yolk on top if you want.

KuriGohan

Total Prep & Cooking Time: 1 hour 45 minutes

Yields: 5 servings

Nutrition Facts: Calories: 264 | Carbs: 57g | Protein: 4.5g | Fat: 0.6g | Fiber: 1.8g

Ingredients:

- One tablespoon of sake
- A quarter cup of sweet rice
- Two cups of short-grain rice (uncooked, Japanese style)
- 20-25 units of chestnuts
- One tsp. of kosher salt
- 2.5 cups of water

For toppings:

- Kosher salt
- Black sesame seeds (toasted)

Method:

1. Wash the rice thoroughly and then allow it to soak in water for half an hour. After that, drain the rice for about fifteen minutes.

2. Boil water in a medium-sized pot. Add the chestnuts. Cover the pot and once boiling starts, put off the flame and keep the pot covered for half an hour. Then, drain them.

3. Peel the chestnut shells and then keep them soaked in water for about ten minutes.

4. Take a heavy bottom pot and in it, add the water, rice, salt, and sake. Lastly, add the chestnuts. Boil the rice and once it boils, keep the flame at low and keep the rice covered for about fifteen minutes. Allow the rice to steam after that for about ten minutes or so. Using a rice paddle, fluff the rice.

5. Sprinkle sesame seeds and salt on top before serving.

MameGohan

Total Prep & Cooking Time: 1 hour and 10 minutes

Yields: 4 servings

Nutrition Facts: Calories: 246 | Carbs: 48g | Protein: 6g | Fat: 1g | Fiber: 0g

Ingredients:

- One kombu
- Half a tablespoon of sake
- Two-third of a cup of green peas, rinsed and drained
- Two cups of Japanese short-grain rice, rinsed and drained
- Half a teaspoon of Kosher salt

Method:

1. Boil two cups of water with half a teaspoon of salt in a medium-size saucepan. Add in the green peas and let it cook for four minutes, so that they are soft yet firm. Turn off the heat and allow it to cool down in the cooking water.

2. After they cool down, pour one cup of the cooking liquid and reserve it for later use.

3. Add the drained rice in a rice cooker bowl and then add the cup of the reserved liquid. Add sake, salt, and kombu. Add in the required extra water and start cooking the rice.

4. Discard the kombu once the rice is cooked.

5. Then, add in the peas and stir to mix it with the rice. Transfer the rice into an airtight container and serve it whenever you like.

Matsutake Gohan

Total Prep & Cooking Time: 1 hour 10 minutes

Yields: Six servings

Nutrition Facts: Calories: 50 | Crabs: 6g | Protein: 2g | Fat: 1g | Fiber: 1g

Ingredients:

- Three cups of Japanese, cooked rice (the cups must be of the size of rice cooker cups)
- Two and a half cups of dashi
- Seven ounces of mushrooms (matsutake)
- Mitsuba to garnish (this is Japanese parsley)

For the seasonings:

- One tablespoon of sake
- Three tablespoons of soy sauce
- Two tablespoons of mirin

Method:

1. Thoroughly wash the rice under running water and then drain the water.

2. Clean the mushrooms of any dirt with a clean towel (avoid washing them). Trim off its stalks. Slice them vertically into one-eighth-inch pieces.

3. Add the seasonings – sake, soy sauce, and mirin) and the rice into a cooker and pour some dashi until it comes to three cups measurement.

4. Form a layer of the mushroom on the rice layer and start to cook. It is better to soak the rice for thirty minutes before putting them into the rice cooker.

5. After you have prepared the rice, take them out— place on a serving plate and mix, tossing them gently and garnish with mitsuba.

Mini Okonomiyaki

Total Prep & Cooking Time: 55 minutes

Yields: Twelve servings

Nutrition Facts: Calories: 570 | Carbs: 23g | Protein: 14g | Fat: 10g | Fiber: 7.2g

Ingredients:

- Two large-sized zucchini (grated coarsely)
- Two-third cups of flour (plain)
- Two eggs (beaten lightly)
- Kewpie mayonnaise
- Two tbsps. each of
- Barbeque sauce
- Olive oil
- Ginger (Japanese pickled)
- One tbsp. of grated onion
- One tsp. of baking powder

- Togarashi (optional)

Method:

1. Take a bowl and add onion and the grated zucchini along with a tsp. of salt to it. Toss well and allow it to sit for about twenty minutes. It will make the veggies lose the extra water. You will have to discard this water later.

2. Take another bowl and fill it with the baking powder and flour. Then add eggs and about two tablespoons of water (cold) and add the seasonings. Whisk the contents slowly to form a thickened and smooth paste. Put the zucchini mixture and combine well.

3. Place a pan over moderate heat and add oil to it. After the oil starts to boil, add the batter with the help of a tablespoon and cook them for three minutes (each side). Cook thoroughly to bring golden brown tinge on each of them. Repeat the same with the remaining batter.

4.   Place the pancakes on a serving plate and then top with barbeque sauce, togarashi, and the pickled ginger strips dipped in mayonnaise. Enjoy it.

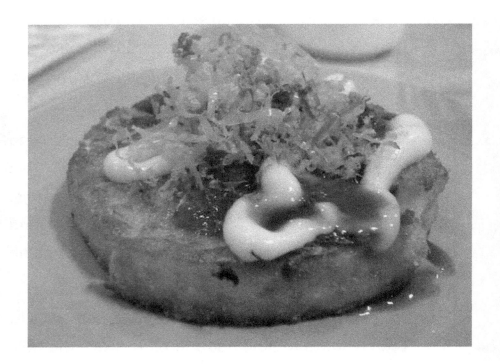

Chapter 2: Vegetable Recipes

Kabocha Gratin

Total Prep & Cooking Time: 1 hour 15 minutes

Yields: 8 servings

Nutrition Facts: Calories: 273 | Carbs: 31g | Protein: 7g | Fat: 13g | Fiber: 2.5g

Ingredients:

- One tablespoon of unsalted butter
- Half a cup of Gruyere cheese
- A quarter cup of Japanese breadcrumbs
- One garlic clove
- Half a unit each of
- Onion
- Kabocha

- 1.5 tablespoons each of
- Miso
- Extra-virgin olive oil
- Freshly ground black pepper
- Kosher salt
- One cup of water
- One package each of
- Shimeji mushrooms
- King oyster mushrooms

For the white sauce:
- 3.3 cups of whole milk
- Half a cup of all-purpose flour
- Four tablespoons of unsalted butter
- One-eighth teaspoon of white pepper powder
- A quarter teaspoon of freshly grated nutmeg
- Kosher salt

For garnishing – parsley or chives

Method:

1.   Remove the pith and seeds of the kabocha and microwave it for a couple of minutes. Peel the skin and cut wedges. Make small chunks about an inch in size.

2.   Slice both garlic and onion in thin strips.

3.   The bottom of the Shimeji mushrooms will have to be discarded, and you can separate the pieces of mushrooms with the help of your hands.

4.   Take the oyster mushrooms and slice them into pieces of about twoinches each.

For making the white sauce:

1.   Melt the butter on low flame in a large pot and then mix the flour in it. Brown the flour and keep stirring for a couple of minutes.

2.   Then, add the milk gradually and keep stirring so that no lumps are formed in the sauce.

3.   Season with nutmeg, white pepper, and kosher salt.

4.   Keep stirring and cook the sauce for about fifteen minutes, and by the end of it, the sauce will become thickened.

For cooking the kabocha:

1.   Heat the oil in a frying pan and then sauté the onion and garlic.

2.   After that, add both the shimeji and oyster mushrooms and cook for about four minutes.

3.   Once they become soft, add the miso. Stir properly.

4.   Then, add a cup of water and the kabocha and allow the mixture to steam. Keep the pan covered and cook for approximately ten minutes.

For assembling:

1.   Now, add the white sauce to the kabocha and season with black pepper and salt if it tastes bland.

2.   Grease your baking dish and then transfer this mixture into it.

3.   Spread grated Gruyere cheese on top and also add some breadcrumbs.

4. Bake the prepared dish for about five minutes at 500 degrees F, and the top should become golden brown.

5. Once done, remove from the oven and cool it for five minutes. Before serving, sprinkle some chives on top.

Daigaku Imo

Total Prep & Cooking Time: 50 minutes

Yields: 4 servings

Nutrition Facts: Calories: 184 | Carbs: 0g | Protein: 0g | Fat: 6g | Fiber: 0g

Ingredients:

- 11 ounces of Satsumaimo or Japanese sweet potatoes
- Five tablespoons of sugar
- Three tablespoons of canola oil
- One teaspoon of black sesame seeds (toasted)
- A quarter teaspoon each of
- Rice vinegar
- Soy sauce

Method:

1. Without peeling the skin, wash the sweet potatoes.

2. Cut the potatoes diagonally in a unique Japanese technique which is known as Rangiri.

3. Then, take some water in a bowl and soak these cut potatoes in it for fifteen minutes.

4. In the frying pan, add oil, sugar, soy sauce, and rice vinegar, and combine them well but do not heat the pan.

5. Now, use a paper towel to dry the potatoes and place them in the pan.

6. Use a linen cloth to cover the lid of the pan. It will ensure that the droplets of water do not fall into the pan. Place the lid on the pan.

7. If you hear bubbling sounds, turn down the flame. Open the lid after every couple of minutes and keep turning the potatoes. It will take you approximately ten minutes for this process to be over.

8. Before serving, sprinkle some toasted black sesame seeds on top of the sweet potatoes.

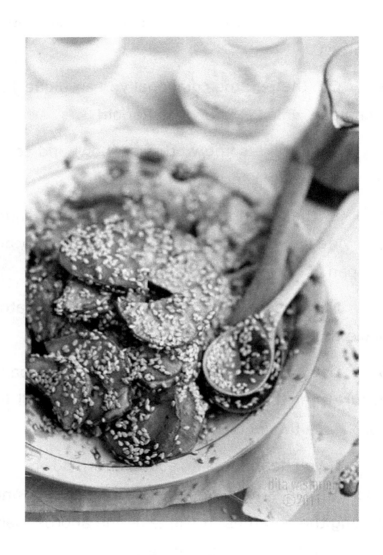

Carrot Ginger Dressing

Total Prep & Cooking Time: 10 minutes

Yields: 6 servings

Nutrition Facts: Calories: 49 | Carbs: 2g | Protein: 0.5g | Fat: 4.5g | Fiber: 0.1g

Ingredients:

- One and a half tablespoons of sugar
- One inch of ginger
- A quarter portion of an onion
- One carrot
- One tablespoon of miso
- A quarter teaspoon of kosher salt
- Half a cup of rice vinegar
- One teaspoon of roasted sesame oil
- Freshly ground black pepper
- A quarter cup of canola oil

Method:

1. Chop the carrot into small pieces after peeling it. Then, chop the onion too.

2. Remove the skin of the ginger and cut small pieces from it.

3. Put everything in the food processor and make a fine puree.

4. Then, add pepper, salt, miso, and sugar.

5. Add rice vinegar, sesame oil, and canola oil.

6. Process the mixture again and make sure it is completely smooth.

7. Serve the dressing over any green salad of your choice.

Edamame Shichimi

Total Prep & Cooking Time: 10 minutes

Yields: 1 serving

Nutrition Facts: Calories: 90 | Carbs: 4.5g | Protein: 6.7g | Fat: 3.4g | Fiber: 0.1g

Ingredients:

- 1 lb. of frozen edamame
- One tbsp. of sesame oil (toasted)
- 3-4 tbsps. of kosher salt (this is specifically for boiling the edamame)
- 2-3 tsps. of shichimi togarashi
- One tsp. of kosher salt

Method:

1. Follow the directions mentioned on the package for preparing the edamame. Drain and pour them in a bowl.
2. Add the rest of the ingredients.
3. Toss well and taste if the seasonings are alright.
4. If needed, add a bit more kosher salt.

Hijiki No Nimono

Total Prep & Cooking Time: 50 minutes

Yields: 4 servings

Nutrition Facts: Calories: 124 | Carbs: 19g | Protein: 2g | Fat: 7g | Fiber: 1g

Ingredients:

- Two aburaage
- Two cups of dashi
- Four cups of water
- Half a cup of hijiki seaweed (dried)
- Three ounces each of
- Carrot
- Konnyaku
- 1.3 ounces of lotus root (pre-boiled)
- One-third cup of shelled edamame
- One tablespoon of canola oil

For the seasonings:

- Four tablespoons each of
- Soy sauce
- Mirin
- Two tablespoons of sugar

Method:

1. Take four cups of water in a bowl and soak the dried hijiki in it for at least half an hour. Use a fine sieve to drain.

2. In a saucepan, boil some water and then pour the boiling water over the aburaage. Slice the aburaage into thin slices.

3. In a small pot, add the konnyaku and water and boil them for about three minutes.

4. Julienne the carrots and also make thin slices from the lotus root.

5. In a medium-sized pot, heat the oil. Add the lotus root and carrots, and cook them.

6. After that, add the hijiki, aburaage, and the konnyaku too. Mix everything properly. Now, add the dashi and bring the mixture to a boil.

7. Once it starts boiling, add the seasonings and cover the pot—Cook for about half an hour.

8. Add the edamame. Cook until the sauce has reduced and then serve.

Okra Ohitashi

Total Prep Time: 15 minutes

Yields: 3 servings

Nutrition Facts: Calories: 50 | Carbs: 3.6g | Protein: 1g | Fat: 0.2g | Fiber: 2g

Ingredients:

- Dried bonito flakes
- Half teaspoon kosher salt
- Ten okras

For the marinade:

- Two tablespoons each of
- Mirin
- Usukuchi soy sauce
- One cup dashi

Method:

1. At first, remove the tail end of the okras. Then peel off the hard portion present around the okra end.

2. Boil some water. On the other hand, sprinkle kosher salt over the okras. It removes the bitterness and also brightens the color.

3. Add the okras into the boiling water and allow it to blanch for about one to two minutes.

4. Drain the water and put the okras in iced water, and allow them to cool. After cooling, remove them from water and squeeze out the excess water.

5. Take a small saucepan and add mirin. Allow the alcohol to evaporate for about one to two minutes.

6. When the alcohol smell disappears, add the soy sauce and dashi. Bring it to a boil, turn off the heat, and keep it aside.

7. Place the okras in a glass baking dish. Pour the marinade into the dish while it's still warm. Leave it for 1 to 2 hours at room temperature.

8. Take a plate, place the okras, drizzle a little marinade, and lastly, sprinkle some dried bonito flakes before serving.

Japanese Pickled Cabbage

Total Prep & Cooking Time: 2 hours 10 minutes

Yields: Four servings

Nutrition Facts: Calories: 45 | Carbs: 8.5g | Protein: 2.4g | Fat: 0.2g | Fiber: 4.7g

Ingredients:

- Half a head of cabbage (ten ounces)
- One chili pepper (red and dried)
- One and a quarter teaspoon of salt
- Half a cucumber (two ounces)
- One dried kelp Kombu (1-inch x3-inch)

For the toppings:

- Soy sauce
- White seeds of sesame (toasted)

Method:

1. Remove the core of cabbage and slice into two-inch pieces.

2. Chop cucumber into half, vertically slice the halves, and then cut the pieces diagonally.

3. Slice the chili into rings, and it is better if you remove the seeds to make the dish less spicy.

4. Roast the Kombu to make them tender and then slice them.

5. Take a plastic bag, fill with the ingredients, and add the salt.

6. Mix the salt with ingredients to coat them properly and close the bag tightly, removing the air.

7. Press the bag so that it touches the pickle and then store it in the refrigerator for three hours.

8. Take out the bag and drain out excess water from the pickled cabbage.

9. Pour some soy sauce and few sesame seeds and enjoy.

Chapter 3: Poultry Recipes

Chicken Teriyaki

Total Prep Time: 55 minutes

Yields: 2 servings

Nutrition Facts: Calories: 130 | Carbs: 5g | Protein: 18g | Fat: 4g | Fiber: 1g

Ingredients:

- One teaspoon canola oil
- Two tablespoons sake
- One tablespoon canola oil
- Ground black pepper
- Salt
- One pound of chicken thighs (skin-on and boneless)
- One-fourth onion

- One inch of ginger

For the teriyaki sauce:

- Two tablespoons each of
- Water
- Soy sauce
- One tablespoon each of
- Sugar
- Mirin
- Sake

Method:

1. Take a bowl and grate some ginger. Add in some juice. Then grate the onion and add to the bowl.

2. Take a separate bowl and add in the sake, mirin, sugar, soy sauce, and water for making the teriyaki sauce.

3. With the help of a fork, prick each side of the chicken, so that the flavor gets nicely absorbed.

4.   Cut out the excess fat and skin. Season it with some salt and pepper.

5.   Take a non-stick pan over medium flame, add one tablespoon of oil, and heat it. Put the chicken keeping the skin side down.

6.   Flip the chicken when the skin turns golden brown. Then add in sake.

7.   Cover and cook for about 8 to 10 minutes over medium-low heat.

8.   Transfer the chicken on a plate and remove the excess oil from the pan.

9.   Heat one teaspoon of oil on the same pan and again place the chicken keeping the skin side down.

10.   Add the prepared sauce and cook until it gets reduced to half.

11.   Turn off the heat and cut the chicken into pieces. Drizzle some sauce over it and serve.

Teba Shio

Total Prep & Cooking Time: 40 minutes

Yields: 3 servings

Nutrition Facts: Calories: 150 | Carbs: 2g | Protein: 15g | Fat: 10g | Fiber: 1g

Ingredients:

- One and a half cups of sake
- Two pounds (about sixteen pieces) of chicken wings (drumettes or flats)
- Lemon (optional)
- Shichimi Togarashi (optional)
- Black pepper, freshly ground
- Sea or Kosher salt

Method:

1. Place an aluminum foil on a baking sheet and keep the wire rack on top. Adjust the rack to the middle position.

2. Pour the sake in a large bowl and soak the chicken wings in it for about ten to fifteen minutes. Flip the wings once mid-way.

3. Use a paper towel to pat dry each wing and then keep them on the wire rack with the skin side up.

4. Sprinkle some black pepper and salt on both sides of the wings and place it with the skin side down.

5. Preheat the broiler on medium or high for about three minutes. Cook the wings in the broiler for about ten minutes. Then, take them out and flip them over. Cook for another ten minutes with the skin side up.

6. You can serve with some lemon wedges or shichimi togarashi on the side.

Notes: *You can also bake the wings if you don't have a broiler—Bake in the oven for forty-five minutes at 200 degrees Celsius. The internal temperature of the* *chicken should be 165 degrees Fahrenheit for it to cook properly.*

Oyakodon

Total Prep & Cooking Time: 30 minutes

Yields: 2 servings

Nutrition Facts: Calories: 591 | Carbs: 78.7g | Protein: 42.8g | Fat: 7.6g | Fiber: 1.4g

Ingredients:

- Two large eggs
- Half an onion, thinly sliced
- Two chicken thighs (boneless and skinless), cut diagonally into 1.5-inch pieces
- Three cups of Japanese short-grain rice (cooked), to serve
- One and a half tablespoons each of
- Soy sauce
- Sake
- Mirin
- Half a cup of dashi

- One and a half teaspoons of sugar
- A small bunch of Mitsuba, chopped
- Shichimi Togarashi (optional)

Method:

1. Add the sugar, soy sauce, sake, mirin, and dashi in a bowl and mix them.

2. Oyakodon is typically cooked one serving at a time. You can Oyakodon pan or an eight-inch frying pan.

3. Add the onions in the pan in a single layer and then add in almost half to one-third of the seasoning mixture. Add in half of the chicken thighs and turn the heat to medium and bring the mixture to a boil.

4. When the mixture starts boiling, reduce the heat to medium-low. Remove any scum or foam from the liquid, cover the pan and let it cook for five minutes so that the onions get soft and the chicken is no longer pink.

5. Beat one egg and slowly add it to the onion and chicken. Cover and cook on medium-low until the egg is cooked according to your liking.

6. Before removing from the heat, add in the chopped mitsubi and pour the dish over a bowl of steamed rice.

7. Add a drizzle of the remaining sauce and serve immediately. You can also add Shichimi Togarashi if you want.

Tsukune

Total Prep & Cooking Time: 35 minutes

Yields: 16 meatballs

Nutrition Facts: Calories: 66.4 | Carbs: 4.6g |Protein: 6.4g | Fat: 2g | Fiber: 0.2g

Ingredients:

- One nori sheet, sliced into thin strips
- One teaspoon each of
- Black sesame seeds
- Castor sugar
- Lemon zest
- Ginger, grated
- One tablespoon each of
- White sesame seeds
- Barbecue sauce
- One clove of garlic, grated

- One small onion, grated
- One pound of chicken thighs (skinless), trimmed and chopped
- One egg white

For the sauce:

- Two teaspoons of Worcestershire sauce
- Two tablespoons each of
- Oyster or barbecue sauce
- Tomato sauce

Method:

1. Preheat your oven to 180 degrees Celsius. Line a baking tray with parchment paper.
2. Mix the ingredients for the sauce in a bowl.

3.   Add the chicken, sugar, barbecue sauce, ginger, garlic, onion, and half a teaspoon of salt in a food processor and whiz for a minute to get a smooth and sticky mixture.

4.   Dampen your hands and make balls from the mixture and place them on the prepared baking tray— Bake for about ten minutes.

5.   Take out the tray and brush the meatballs with half of the sauce. Add a sprinkle of sesame seeds and then bake for another ten minutes until they are cooked properly and become golden.

6.   Add sixteen dollops of the sauce on a serving plate and keep the meatballs beside the sauce. Add the nori sheets and serve.

Soboro Don

Total Prep & Cooking Time: 30 minutes

Yields: 2-3 servings

Nutrition Facts: Calories: 164 | Carbs: 13g | Protein: 24g | Fat: 1.4g | Fiber: 3.6g

Ingredients:

For the chicken:

- Two tablespoons of soy sauce
- One tablespoon each of
- Mirin
- Sake
- Canola oil
- One and a half tablespoons of sugar
- One teaspoon of ginger, grated along with its juice
- Half a pound of ground chicken

For the scrambled eggs:

- One tablespoon each of
- Canola oil
- Sugar
- Two large eggs

To serve:

- Beni shoga
- One-fourth of a cup of green peas (defrosted)
- Two servings of Japanese short-grain rice (cooked)

Method:

1. Place a nonstick frying pan over medium heat and heat oil in it. Add in the ground chicken and cook until it's no longer pink. Break it up into small pieces with the help of a wooden spoon.

2.   Add in the soy sauce, mirin, sugar, and sake and continue to break it up into smaller bits. Add in the ginger with its juice when the meat is broken into smaller bits.

3.   Cook the chicken until almost all the liquid has evaporated. Pour it int a bowl and keep aside.

4.   Whisk the eggs and sugar in a small bowl and prepare some long cooking chopsticks.

5.   Place another frying pan over medium-low heat and add oil into it. Add in the whisked egg and break the egg into small pieces with the help of the chopsticks. Transfer it to a bowl once it's cooked.

6.   Add the steamed rice into serving bowls and add the peas, ground chicken, and scrambled egg as a topping. Garnish with pickled ginger and serve.

Chapter 4: Seafood Recipes

Unagi Chazuke

Total Prep & Cooking Time: 15 minutes

Yields: 2 servings

Nutrition Facts: Calories: 626 | Carbs: 91g | Protein: 24g | Fat: 18g | Fiber: 5g

Ingredients:

For Unagi Donburi:

- Two servings of cooked rice (Japanese short-grain)
- Two to three tablespoons of unagi sauce
- One fillet of unagi (about 5.6 ounces), precooked and sliced into half or thirds

For the broth:

- Two teaspoons of konbucha
- Two cups of dashi

For garnish:

- One teaspoon of white sesame seeds, toasted
- One bunch of Mitsuba (optional), chopped
- One scallion or green onion (optional), chopped

Method:

1. Mix the konbucha and dashi in a small saucepan and heat it over medium heat. Stir well. You can add more salt or konbucha according to your taste.

2. Place the unagi pieces on a baking sheet lined with parchment paper. Place it in the middle rack of the oven and broil on high for seven minutes.

3. Remove from oven and brush the unagi sauce over it. Broil for an additional thirty to sixty seconds.

4. Add steamed rice in the serving bowls and brush some unagi sauce on it and place the unagi pieces on top. You can add more unagi sauce if you want.

5. Pour the sauce in the bowl right before serving and add the sesame seeds, mitsuba, and green onions as a garnish.

Kaki Fry

Total Prep & Cooking Time: 30 minutes

Yields: Four servings

Nutrition Facts: Calories: 125 | Carbs: 15g | Protein: 6g | Fat: 4.3g | Fiber: 0g

Ingredients:

- Four cups of green cabbage, shredded
- One cup of Japanese panko breadcrumbs
- Two large eggs, beaten
- One-fourth cup of all-purpose flour
- Canola oil
- Sixteen oysters
- Dash of black pepper and salt
- One bottle of tonkatsu sauce (optional)
- One lemon, cut into wedges (garnish)

Method:

1. Use salted water to clean the oysters and then dry them using paper towels—season with black pepper and salt.

2. Place a medium-sized pot over medium-high heat and add one to two cups of oil into it.

3. Take three separate shallow dishes, and add panko in one, beaten eggs in another, and flour in the last one.

4. Coat the oysters in the flour first, then dip them in eggs, and lastly, coat them with the breadcrumbs.

5. Fry the oysters in the oil when it has reached a temperature of 350 degrees Fahrenheit. Fry for one to two minutes until they turn brown. Flip them once midway. They are done when they start floating in the oil. Transfer them to a dish lined with paper towels to drain the excess oil and keep warm.

6. Serve the oysters along with shredded cabbage and add the lemon wedges as a garnish. You can also serve with tonkatsu or tartar sauce.

Smoked Ocean Trout and Noodles

Total Prep & Cooking Time: 30 minutes

Yields: 4 servings

Nutrition Facts: Calories: 395 | Carbs: 48g | Protein: 22.2g | Fat: 11.4g | Fiber: 4g

Ingredients:

- One tablespoon of canola oil
- One and a half tablespoons of soy sauce
- Three teaspoons of sesame oil
- Two tablespoons of rice vinegar
- One cup of bean sprouts
- One-third of a cup each of
- Mint leaves
- Coriander leaves
- Three spring onions, sliced thinly at an angle

- One Lebanese cucumber, sliced into ribbons
- Two packets of smoked ocean trout (10.5 ounces), skin discarded
- 9.5 ounces of organic somen noodles

Method:

1. Boil water in a large saucepan and cook the somen noodles according to the instructions given on the package. Rinse the noodles under cold water and then drain again.

2. Pour the noodles in a large bowl and sprinkle the fish on the top. Add in the bean sprouts, herbs, spring onions, and cucumber and gently toss everything to combine.

3. Add the rest of the ingredients in a bowl and whisk to mix them. Add this dressing into the bowl of noodles and gently mix them. Top with the remaining dressing and serve.

Miso Butter Snapper

Total Prep & Cooking Time: 30 minutes

Yields: Two servings

Nutrition Facts: Calories: 203 | Carbs: 5g | Protein: 19g | Fat: 10g | Fiber: 0g

Ingredients:

- One tbsp. each of
- Miso paste (white)
- Soy sauce
- Peanut oil
- Skinless fillets of snapper (12.7 ounces)
- Two red chilies (small-sized and sliced thinly)
- Two bunches of broccoli (sliced vertically into halves)
- One tsp. each of
- Sesame oil
- Sesame seeds

- Spring onion to garnish (sliced thinly)
- Mushrooms with trimmed stalks (mixed - enoki and shimeji), approximately 5.29 ounces
- Half a lime juiced
- Softened butter, unsalted (about one ounce)

Method:

1. Set the oven at a temperature of 200 degrees C. Take a baking dish and line its edges with a baking paper.

2. In a bowl, mix the butter and the miso properly—brush the snapper fillets with this paste.

3. Take another bowl and add chili, peanut oil, sesame oil, and soy sauce to it, mixing correctly. Then add the mushrooms, sesame seeds, and broccoli. Toss to coat the veggies well with previously mixed ingredients in the bowl. Take the mixture and then coat the base of the baking dish with it, forming a single layer. Place the snapper on the bed of veggies mixture and then bake for twenty minutes.

4. Take the baking dish out and transfer the fillets to a serving plate. Garnish with lime juice and extra chili along with some scattered spring onion. Enjoy it.

KinmedaiNitsuke

Total Prep & Cooking Time: 30 minutes

Yields: Two servings

Nutrition Facts: Calories: 110 | Carbs: 11g | Protein: 1g | Fat: 0g | Fiber: 0g

Ingredients:

- Half a pound of kinmedai filet (wash them thoroughly under running water and soak the water by dry pat)
- One tablespoon each of
- Rice vinegar
- Sugar
- Two tablespoons each of
- Mirin
- Soy sauce
- One cup of water
- A one-third cup of sake

- Two slices of fresh ginger

Method:

1. Place a medium-sized saucepan over moderate heat. Pour water, add fish fillets, and as the surface turns white, stop cooking. Wash the fish in cold water and keep it aside—Wash off the pan.

2. Place the washed pan over the flame and then add the sake, ginger, soy sauce, and sugar to it. Cook the ingredients in boiling water and then add the fish. Cover the pan with a drop lid and cook over low heat for fifteen minutes. Keep an eye on the pan to check the sauce consistency.

3. Remove the lid and lift the fish filets on a serving plate with care. Drizzle the fish with sauce and serve warm.

Are you enjoying this book? If so, i'd be really happy if you could leave a short review on Amazon, it means a lot to me! Thank you.

Chapter 5: Udon and Soba Noodles Recipes

Curry Udon Noodles

Total Prep & Cooking Time: 40 minutes

Yields: 2 servings

Nutrition Facts: Calories: 340 | Carbs: 47g | Protein: 7g | Fat: 14g | Fiber: 1g

Ingredients:

- One spring onion
- 760ml water
- Four tablespoons of tsuyu soup stock
- Two packets of udon noodles (pre-cooked)
- Half each of
- Carrot

- Potato
- Onion
- Three blocks of Japanese curry roux

Method:

1. Add 360ml of water to a pan. Chop the carrot, potato, and onion into small pieces and add them to the pan.

2. Bring it to a boil. Simmer until the vegetables soften, for about 2o minutes.

3. Add three blocks of curry roux and simmer for ten minutes. Stir continuously until the curry sauce is smooth and thick.

4. Take a separate pan, add 400ml of water, and add four tbsp of tsuyu soup stock for making the noodle soup. Boil it.

5. Boil the udon noodles and drain them after a few minutes in the colander.

6. Take a bowl and place the udon noodles, pour the noodle soup, pour the curry sauce on top. Before serving, garnish with some sliced spring onions.

Kitsune Udon

Total Prep & Cooking Time: 50 minutes

Yields: 2 servings

Nutrition Facts: Calories: 413 | Carbs: 58g | Protein: 10g | Fat: 15.5g | Fiber: 0g

Ingredients:

- Four pouches of Inari Age
- Two servings of udon noodles
- One scallion or green onion, sliced thinly
- One tablespoon each of
- Usukuchi soy sauce
- Mirin
- Two and a quarter cups of dashi
- One teaspoon of sugar
- Half a teaspoon of sea salt or kosher salt
- Shichimi Togarashi (optional)

- Narutomaki (optional), cut into 1/8 inch pieces

For the homemade dashi:

- One and a half cups of katsuobushi
- One kombu
- Two and a half cups of water

Method:

1. You can use store-bought dashi powder or make it on your own. To make the homemade dashi, add the kombu in two and a half cups of water and let it soak for at least thirty minutes. You can also soak it for three hours or up to half a day as it helps bring out the flavor of the kombu.

2. Add the kombu and water into a saucepan and boil it over medium-low heat. Discard the kombu just before the water starts boiling. The dashi will turn bitter and slimy if you keep the kombu in the water for too long while it is boiling.

3. Add in one and a half cups of katsuobushi and boil again. Lower the heat when the dashi is boiling and let

it simmer for fifteen minutes and then turn off the heat. Allow the katsuobushi to sink to the bottom of the pan and then keep it for ten to fifteen minutes. Use a fine-mesh sieve to strain the dashi into a saucepan. Your homemade dashi is now ready.

4. Add the soy sauce, sugar, mirin, dashi, and salt into a saucepan and boil the mixture. Then, cover or turn off the heat and let it simmer.

5. Add the udon noodles into a large pot of water and boil it. Once it gets cooked, transfer it into a strainer and drain all the water.

6. Add the soup and the udon noodles equally into serving bowls and add the shichimi togarashi, green onions, narutomaki, and Inari Age as a garnish.

Momofuku Soy Sauce Eggs, Chili Chicken, and Soba Noodles

Total Prep & Cooking Time: 30 minutes

Yields: 4 servings

Nutrition Facts: Calories: 443.3 | Carbs: 38g | Protein: 40g | Fat: 16g | Fiber: 3g

Ingredients:

- 3.5 ounces of enoki mushrooms, trimmed
- One toasted nori sheet, torn
- 9.5 ounces of soba noodles, cooked and refreshed
- Four eggs, hard-boiled and peeled
- Three cups of chicken stock
- One-third of a cup of white miso paste
- One teaspoon each of
- Ginger, finely grated

- Chili garlic paste
- Four spring onions, thinly sliced and some extra shredded onions for serving
- 7 ounces of chicken, minced
- Two teaspoons of olive oil (extra virgin)
- One cup each of
- Soy sauce
- Rice wine vinegar
- Shichimi togarashi, to serve

Method:

1. Keep the eggs, soy sauce, and vinegar in a non-reactive bowl and chill overnight or for three to four hours.

2. Place a frying pan over high heat and add one teaspoon of oil in it. Then add the minced chicken and cook for five minutes and break the pieces using a wooden spoon. Add in the chili garlic paste when the chicken turns brown and cook for another three to four minutes so that they get brownish. Keep warm.

3. Place a saucepan over medium-low heat and heat the remaining teaspoon of oil in it. Add in the ginger and onions and cook for three to four minutes and occasionally stir so that they get tender. Add in the stock and miso and stir so that the miso dissolves.

4. Divide the nori, soup, and noodles among serving bowls. Add the extra onion, mushroom, halved eggs and mince mixture as a topping. Sprinkle some shichimi togarashi and serve.

Soba Noodle and Broccolini Salad

Total Prep & Cooking Time: 15 minutes

Yields: 2 servings

Nutrition Facts: Calories: 444 | Carbs: 76.4g | Protein: 18.6g | Fat: 11g | Fiber: 3g

Ingredients:

- One avocado, sliced
- Six ounces of soba noodles, cooked and drained
- Two teaspoons each of
- Ginger, finely chopped
- Soy sauce
- One and a half teaspoons of sea salt flakes
- One teaspoon each of
- Mirin
- Wasabi paste

- Peanut oil
- One cup of podded edamame (frozen), thawed
- Two bunches of broccolini (sliced lengthwise)
- Two eggs, boiled and peeled

Method:

1. Boil water in a saucepan and cook the broccolini in it for two minutes so that they turn just soft. Add in the edamame and cook for another minute. Drain the vegetables and keep aside.

2. Prepare the dressing by mixing the mirin, wasabi, peanut oil, and soy sauce in a bowl. Keep it aside.

3. Prepare the ginger salt by rubbing the ginger and salt together with your fingers.

4. Add the avocado, broccolini, and soba noodles in a large bowl and add a drizzle of the dressing. Slice the boiled egg into quarters and add it on top of the noodles. Add a sprinkle of ginger salt and serve.

Soba, Prawn, and Lemongrass Soup

Total Prep & Cooking Time: 1 hour and 20 minutes

Yields: 4 servings

Nutrition Facts: Calories: 180.6 | Carbs: 35g | Protein: 20g | Fat: 0.3g | Fiber: 2.3g

Ingredients:

- Six ounces of dried soba noodles
- 10.5 ounces of king prawns (medium-sized), peeled and deveined with the tails intact
- Eight cups of chicken stock
- 6-inch piece of lemongrass (only the white part), cut in half lengthwise
- 1.5-inch of ginger, thinly sliced
- Two eschalots, thinly sliced
- Two teaspoons each of

- Sesame oil
- Soy sauce
- Two green shallots, thinly sliced
- One red chili, thinly sliced
- One teaspoon each of
- Sesame seeds
- Rice vinegar
- Mirin

Method:

1. Place a large saucepan over medium-high heat and heat some sesame oil in it. Add in the ginger and eschalots and cook for three to four minutes so that the eschalots get tender. Add in the chicken stock and lemongrass and boil the mixture. Lower the heat to low and let it simmer for thirty-five to forty minutes.

2. Add in the prawns and cook for another two to three minutes. Then, add the vinegar, mirin, soy, and noodles and stir.

3. Pour the soup into serving bowls and top with green shallots, chili, and sesame seeds.

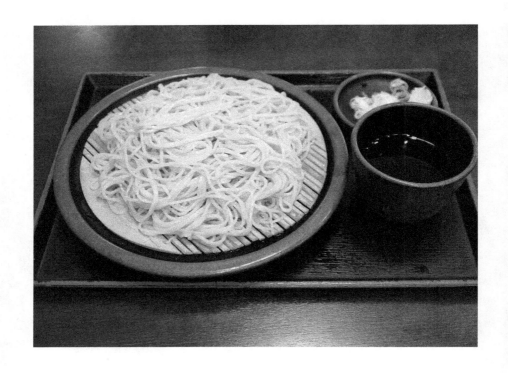

Chapter 6: Tofu Recipes

Goya Champuru

Total Prep & Cooking Time: 40 minutes

Yields: 2 servings

Nutrition Facts: Calories: 118 | Carbs: 2g | Protein: 8g | Fat: 7g | Fiber: 1g

Ingredients:

- One tablespoon of soy sauce
- Canola oil
- Two large eggs, beaten
- Six pieces of pork belly, sliced onto one-inch pieces
- Fourteen ounces of tofu (medium-firm), torn into bite-size pieces

- One bitter melon, cut in half lengthwise, deseeded, and sliced into 1/8-inch pieces
- Freshly ground black pepper
- Kosher or sea salt

For the Katsuo Dashi:

- One-fourth of a cup of boiling water
- Three tablespoons of katsuobushi

Method:

1. Add a teaspoon of salt on the bitter melon and mix it properly. Allow it to rest or ten minutes and then rinse with water and drain properly.

2. In the meantime, drain the excess water from the tofu. Wrap it in a paper towel and keep a heavy object on top of it for about ten minutes. You can sandwich the tofu in between two flat trays and place a marble mortar on top of it.

3. Add one-fourth cup of boiling water in a measuring cup along with the katsuoboshi. Set it aside

until you're ready to cook and let it steep. Strain the liquid and throw away the katsuobushi. Keep it aside for now.

4.   Heat one tablespoon of oil in a large frying pan and add the tofu in it. Cook them until they turn brown and then transfer to a plate.

5.   Add another tablespoon of oil in the pan and add in the bitter melon with some salt. Stir fry and then transfer onto a plate.

6.   Heat half teaspoon of oil and add in the pork belly. Add the black pepper and salt and stir fry until they turn golden brown.

7.   Transfer the tofu and bitter melon back into the pan along with the dashi and soy sauce. Toss to mix everything while the liquid evaporates.

8.   Add the eggs into the pan and shake the pan to cook the egg. Turn off the heat and serve when the egg is no longer runny.

Hiyayakko

Total Prep & Cooking Time: 5 minutes

Yields: 4 servings

Nutrition Facts: Calories: 128 | Carbs: 4g | Protein: 14g | Fat: 5g | Fiber: 3g

Ingredients:

- Two tablespoons of soy sauce
- Two teaspoons of grated ginger
- One scallion or green onion, thinly sliced
- Four tablespoons of katsuobushi
- Fourteen ounces of chilled tofu (soft or silken)

Method:

1. Wrap a paper towel around the tofu and drain it for ten to fifteen minutes. Cut it into four to six pieces once the liquid is drained.

2. Place the pieces of tofu on a serving dish and top with ginger, green onions, or any of your favorite toppings.

3. Add a drizzle of soy sauce or any other sauce on top and serve.

Tofu Pizza

Total Prep & Cooking Time: 25 minutes

Yields: 2 servings

Nutrition Facts: Calories: 113 | Carbs: 13g | Protein: 6g | Fat: 4g | Fiber: 1g

Ingredients:

- One cup of mozzarella cheese, grated
- One-fourth cup of cornstarch or potato starch
- One tomato, thinly sliced
- Two mushrooms, thinly sliced
- Three slices of ham, cut into thin strips
- One block of tofu, cut in half
- Two to four basil leaves
- Two to three tablespoons of ketchup
- Freshly ground black pepper
- Half a teaspoon of salt

- Parsley (for garnishing)

Method:

1. Wrap each half of the tofu in paper towels and keep it under a plate. Place a heavy object on the top to help drain the tofu. Keep aside for fifteen minutes.

2. Add the cornstarch on a plate and season with salt and pepper. Coat all sides of the tofu with the seasoned cornstarch.

3. Place an oven-safe skillet over medium-high heat and heat oil in it. Place the tofu in it and cook until the bottom turns golden brown and crispy. Turn it over and cook the other side.

4. Add the ketchup on the top and spread evenly. Then add the tomato, basil, ham, cheese, and mushrooms on the top.

5. Insert the pan in the oven and broil for five to seven minutes so that the cheese melts.

6. Serve hot.

Chapter 7: Sushi Recipes

Dragon Rolls

Total Prep & Cooking Time: One hour

Yields: 4 rolls

Nutrition Facts: Calories: 71 | Carbs: 5.8g | Protein: 4.6g | Fat: 3.2g | Fiber: 0.5g

Ingredients:

- Two tablespoons of Tobiko
- Eight pieces of shrimp tempura
- Two cups of sushi rice (seasoned and cooked)
- Two nori sheets, cut in half crosswise
- Two avocados, cut in half
- One Japanese or Persian cucumber, cut lengthwise into quarters
- Unagi (optional)

- Half a lemon(optional)

Toppings:

- Black sesame seeds, toasted
- Unagi sauce
- Spicy mayo

Tezu:

- Two teaspoons of rice vinegar
- One-fourth cup of water

Method:

1. Peel the skin of the avocado and slice it widthwise. Press the slices gently so that they elongate evenly and reach the length of the nori sheet.

2. Keep half of the nori sheet on the bamboo mat with the shiny side down. Wet your fingertips with the tezu. After that, evenly spread half a cup of the sushi rice on top of the sheet.

3. Flip it over carefully and add the tobiko, cucumber pieces, unagi (optional), and shrimp tempura on the bottom edge of the sheet.

4. Roll over the bamboo mat and squeeze tightly.

5. Add the avocado on top of the sushi roll with the help of a knife.

6. Gently wrap the avocado slices around the sushi roll with the help of a plastic wrap and then cut the roll into eight pieces.

7. Remove the plastic before serving and add tobiko, spicy mayo on top of the sushi roll. Sprinkle some black sesame seeds and enjoy.

California Rolls

Total Prep & Cooking Time: 1 hour

Yields: 8 rolls

Nutrition Facts: Calories: 349 | Carbs: 38g | Protein: 7.8g | Fat: 19g | Fiber: 3.2g

Ingredients:

- One-fourth cup of white sesame seeds, toasted
- Eight nori sheets
- Half a lemon
- Two avocados, peeled, pitted, and cut into quarter-inch slices
- Half of an English cucumber, cut into long strips
- Six tablespoons of Japanese mayonnaise
- Nine ounces of crab meat, cooked
- Six cups of sushi rice, seasoned and cooked
- Tobiko

Tezu:

- Two teaspoons of rice vinegar
- One-fourth cup of water

Method:

1. Mix the crab meat with the mayonnaise to prepare the filling.

2. Cut off one-third of the nori sheet and save it for later. Place the remaining two-thirds of the sheet on top of a bamboo mat (shiny side down) lined with plastic wrap.

3. Dip your fingertips in the tezu. Then, evenly spread one cup of the sushi rice on top of the nori sheet. Sprinkle the tobiko or sesame seeds on top.

4. Flip the nori sheet carefully and add the avocado, cucumber, and crab meat on the bottom end of the nori sheet.

5. Roll the mat into a tight cylinder so that the fillings are tucked in firmly.

6. Cut the roll into pieces with the help of a sharp knife and serve.

Cucumber Wrapped Sushi

Total Prep & Cooking Time: 1 hour and 15 minutes

Yields: 15 sushis

Nutrition Facts: Calories: 40.3 | Carbs: 1.2g | Protein: 7g | Fat: 1.1g | Fiber: 0.2g

Ingredients:

- Three to four cups of sushi rice, seasoned and cooked
- Two Japanese cucumbers, cut into long and thin strips

Toppings:

- Ten Sashimi-grade shrimp
- Four tablespoons of Ikura
- Four ounces each of
- Sashimi-grade tuna
- Sashimi-grade yellowtail

- Sashimi-grade salmon

For garnishing:

- Kaiware radish sprouts
- One lemon
- One scallion or green onion
- Ten Shiso leaves

Method:

1. Place the shiso leaves on a plate and keep a cookie cutter on top of it. Add the sushi rice inside the cookie cutter and stuff it in about halfway. Then, gently remove the cutter and use a strip of cucumber to roll the sushi cylinder. Create slits at the ends of the cucumber strips so that you can interlock them around the sushi.

2. Add your favorite topping on each sushi roll and garnish with Daikon radish sprouts and lemon. Serve immediately.

Saba Oshizushi

Total Prep & Cooking Time: 40 minutes

Yields: 2 servings

Nutrition Facts: Calories: 135 | Carbs: 20.6g | Protein: 32.9g | Fat: 29g | Fiber: 2.5g

Ingredients:

- Four tablespoons each of rice vinegar
- Six shiso leaves
- One fillet of frozen marinated mackerel (defrosted overnight)
- Two cups of Japanese short-grain rice (uncooked)
- One teaspoon of sea salt or Kosher salt
- Two tablespoons of sugar

Method:

1. Cook the rice in a rice cooker. Fluff it up with a paddle or rice scooper once the rice has cooked properly.

2. Take hangiri or sushi oke and moisten it so that the rice won't stick to it. Add the cooked rice into it and spread it outevenly.

3. When the rice is still warm, add the rice vinegar into it and mix it with the rice with a rice paddle. Cool the rice in the meantime, so that it doesn't turn mushy.

4. Cut the defrosted mackerel fillets into half lengthwise and butterfly them from the cut edge. Repeat with the other half.

5. Make the tezu with water and a tablespoon of rice vinegar and wet your hands with it.

6. Take an Oshibako mold and moisten it with the tezu.

7. Add the mackerel fillet (skin side down), followed by the shiso leaves, and lastly, add the rice. Fill the mold just above the rim and press down firmly with the top piece.

8. Remove the finished oshizushi from the mold and cut it into pieces with a sharp knife. Clean the mold and moisten it once again before preparing the next batch.

9. Add pickled ginger as a garnish and serve.

Chapter 8: Soup Recipes

Tonjiru

Total Prep & Cooking Time: 40 minutes

Yields: 4 servings

Nutrition Facts: Calories: 121 | Carbs: 5.3g | Protein: 5.5g | Fat: 8.4g | Fiber: 2g

Ingredients:

For the soup:

- Seven ounces of tofu (medium-firm), cut into half-inch cubes
- One teaspoon of ginger, peeled and grated
- One piece of aburaage, cut into thin slices
- One Negi, sliced diagonally
- 4.5 ounces of konnyaku, cut into thin rectangular pieces

- Four ounces of carrots, peeled and cut into thin slices
- Nine ounces of daikon radish, peeled and cut into 1/8 inch slices
- One onion, cut into thin slices
- Eight ounces of Taro, peeled and cut into 1/3 inch slices
- Four ounces of gobo
- Ten ounces of pork belly, sliced into one-inch pieces

For making the soup:
- Six tablespoons of miso
- Six cups of dashi
- One tablespoon of roasted sesame oil

To garnish:
- Shichimi togarashi (optional)
- One scallion or green onion, cut into thin small rounds

Method:

1. Use the back of your knife to scrape the outer skin of the gobo. Make a one-inch deep cross incision at one end of the gobo.

2. Rub one-fourth teaspoon of salt over the cut konnyaku pieces and leave it for five minutes. Then, add it to boiling water and cook for two to three minutes.

3. Heat sesame oil in a large pot over medium heat and add the pork belly into it. Stir fry the pork until it's no longer pink. Add the onion, carrot, and daikon and stir. Add in the Taro, gobo, Negi, aburaage, and konnyaku. Add enough dashi to cover the ingredients and stir.

4. Close the lid and bring the mixture to a boil. Decrease the heat when boiling and remove the fat and scum from the soup.

5. Cover the pot and simmer for ten to fifteen minutes so that the root vegetables get soft.

6. Add the miso right before serving to enhance the flavor of the soup. Then, tear the tofu into pieces and add them into the soup along with the ginger.

7. Add some green onions on the top and serve.

Matsutake Clear Soup

Total Prep & Cooking Time: 20 minutes

Yields: 2 servings

Nutrition Facts: Calories: 241 | Carbs: 21g | Protein: 4.1g | Fat: 16g | Fiber: 2g

Ingredients:

- Four stalks of Mitsuba
- 5.1 ounces of tofu (soft or silken), cut into small cubes
- One matsutake mushroom, cut into thin slices
- Yuzu zest
- Four Temari Fu (optional)

For the dashi:

- 0.4 ounces of katsuobushi
- 0.2 ounces of kombu
- Two cups of water

For seasoning:

- Two teaspoons each of
- Soy sauce
- Mirin
- One tablespoon of sake
- Half a teaspoon of salt

Method:

1. Use a damp towel to clean the matsutake mushrooms. Remember that you shouldn't wash them. Cut off and remove a thin slice of the stem of the mushroom with the help of a knife and cut into thin slices.

2. Clean the dashi kombu using a clean cloth. The white powdery substance increases the flavor of the umami in the dashi, so leave it on. Don't wash the dashi.

3. Take water in a medium-sized saucepan and add the kombu in it. Slowly heat in on medium-low heat.

You can also soak it in water for up to half a day if you have time. Soaking it helps bring out the kombu's flavor naturally.

4. Add in the katsuobushi when it starts boiling. Allow it to simmer for thirty seconds and then turn off the heat.

5. Line a sieve with a paper towel and keep it over a bowl. Strain the dashi into the bowl. Twist and squeeze the paper towel and release any excess dashi into the bowl.

6. Add the dashi into a saucepan and boil it. Add in the soy sauce, mirin, sake, and salt. Then, add in the tofu and the mushrooms and cook for two to three minutes.

7. Add the temari fu in water to allow it to hydrate. When it gets soft, squeeze out the water and transfer it into a serving bowl.

8. Take two mitsuba stalks and tie them into a knot. Before serving, add the two knotted mitsuba stalks into the soup.

Tofu and Japanese Pumpkin soup

Total Prep & Cooking Time: 45 minutes

Yields: 4 servings

Nutrition Facts: Calories: 144.6 | Carbs: 20g | Protein: 11g | Fat: 3g | Fiber: 4g

Ingredients:

- 7 ounces of mixed mushrooms, trimmed and sliced
- 3 ounces of baby spinach
- 3.5 ounces of tofu (silken firm), cut into half-inch cubes
- Two tablespoons of mirin
- One-fourth cup of soy sauce
- Two sachets of instant dashi powder (0.7 ounces)
- 35 ounces of butternut pumpkin, peeled and cut into half-inch cubes

- Sesame seeds (toasted) and sesame oil, to serve

Method:

1. Add six cups of slightly salted water into a saucepan placed over medium heat.

2. Add in the pumpkin and simmer for ten to fifteen minutes so that they just soft. Add in the mirin, soy sauce, dashi powder, and tofu and let it simmer for five minutes.

3. Add the mushrooms and spinach and cook for thirty seconds so that they wilt. Take it away from the heat.

4. Pour the soup into serving bowls and drizzle some sesame oil and top with toasted sesame seeds.

Champon

Total Prep & Cooking Time: 40 minutes

Yields: Two servings

Nutrition Facts: Calories: 522 | Carbs: 93g | Protein: 23g | Fat: 18g | Fiber: 3.4g

Ingredients:

For preparing the soup:

- Two cups of chicken broth
- One tablespoon each of
- Sake
- Soy sauce
- A quarter cup of milk (whole)
- Half a teaspoon of salt
- One cup of dashi
- One teaspoon of sugar
- One-eighth teaspoon of pepper powder (white)

For preparing meat and the seafood:

- Two ounces each of
- Pork belly (two slices)
- Squid
- One teaspoon of soy sauce
- Two and a half ounces of shrimp
- One tablespoon of sake

For the vegetables and other ingredients:

- Six pieces of ear mushrooms (dried wood)
- A quarter of an onion
- One ounce of snow pea
- Four ounces of bean sprouts
- Black pepper (ground freshly)
- Eleven ounces of champon noodles
- Two inches of carrot
- Five ounces of cabbage

- A one-third of fish cake (kamaboko)
- One tablespoon of roasted sesame oil
- One-eighth teaspoon of salt

Method:

1. Add the chicken broth (two cups) and the dashi (one cup) in a pot. Combine them with a spoon. To this mixture, add soy sauce, sake, and granulated sugar (one teaspoon). Allow them to cook.

2. Once they start boiling, add the milk and white pepper.

3. Slice the pork belly into pieces of one inch. Add soy sauce and sake (each of one teaspoon) to it.

4. Place the shrimp, squid, and two teaspoons of sake in the bowl. Set the bowl aside for about five minutes.

5. Slice the squid by moving the knife diagonally (make parallel lines). You can make simple incisions on the flesh.

6. Take another bowl and add then the mushrooms. Pour enough water in the bowl to immerse the

mushroom pieces. Rehydrate the mushrooms to soften them and then squeeze out the extra water. Slice into pieces.

7. Make thin slabs of the carrot and then half the slices vertically. Chop the onion. Discarding the core of cabbage, cut them into cubes. Cut the snow peas into halves after removing the strings from them. Make thin slices of the kamaboko fish.

8. Place a wok over moderate to high heat and add sesame oil to it. After the oil starts to boil, add pork belly pieces and cook until they brown. Add the squid and the shrimp pieces to it and cook until they become opaque.

9. Stir in carrot and onion. Add mushroom and cabbage, and keep stirring for one minute. Stir in the bean sprouts, the snow peas, and fish—Cook for an additional minute. Sprinkle pepper and then toss them to combine. Add the soup to the wok and then adjust the salt by tasting it.

10. Prepare the noodles: Cut the packet, take the noodles out, and then separate them, place a large pan over a moderate flame, and pour

water. Put the noodle strips in it—Cook noodles and place in a bowl.

11. Top the noodles with the soup and other toppings. Serve them warm.

Chapter 9: Snacks & Dessert Recipes

Mochi Ice Cream

Total Prep Time: 1 hour 3 minutes

Yields: 12 pieces

Nutrition Facts: Calories: 80 | Carbs: 14g | Protein: 1g | Fat: 2.5g | Fiber: 0g

Ingredients:

- Ice cream
- Half cup cornstarch/ potato starch
- One-fourth cup sugar
- Three-fourth cup each of
- Water
- Shiratamako

Method:

1. Scoop out the ice cream into silicon/aluminum cupcake liners. Freeze them.

2. Combine sugar and shiratamako in a medium bowl. Whisk together. Add water and mix well.

3. Cover the bowl with plastic and put it inside the microwave. Heat it for one minute on high heat. Bring it out, stir, and again cook for one minute. Again stir it, cover it, and then cook for another 30 seconds.

4. Cover the work surface using parchment paper. Sprinkle a generous amount of potato starch.

5. Place the cooked mochi and again sprinkle some potato starch on top of it.

6. Spread the mochi to form a thin layer using a rolling pin.

7. Transfer the mochi to a baking sheet along with the parchment paper.

8. Refrigerate for about fifteen minutes.

9. Take it out and cut into 7 to 8 circles.

10. Shed the excess potato starch. Take a plate, place a plastic wrap, then place the mochi and wrapper. Again place a plastic wrapper and repeat the process for all the wrappers. Roll the rest of the mochi dough into a ball. Form a flat and thin layer. Cut out more circle wrappers from it.

11. Place one plastic wrap sheet, on the working surface, along with the mochi on top. Place the frozen ice cream ball on the top of the mochi layer. Wrap the ice cream ball and pinch the layer to close the corners.

12. Wrap them with plastic and place them in a cupcake pan and keep them in the freezer. After a few hours, they will be ready to serve.

Anmitsu

Total Prep Time: 30 minutes

Yields: 6 servings

Nutrition Facts: Calories: 125 | Carbs: 30g | Protein: 1g | Fat: 0g | Fiber: 0g

Ingredients:

- Kuromitsu
- Kiwis
- Banana
- Strawberries
- Six scoops of vanilla ice cream or green tea ice cream
- Six tablespoons of Anko
- One batch each of
- ShiratamaDango
- Agar-agar jelly

Method:

1. Prepare the shiratamaDango and agar-agar jelly beforehand.

2. Cut the fruits into small pieces.

3. Divide the ice cream, red bean paste, shiratamadango, fruits, and agar-agar jelly evenly into separate bowls.

4. Serve along with kuromitsu.

Fruit Jelly

Total Prep & Cooking Time: 6 hours 13 minutes

Yields: 9 fruit jelly cubes

Nutrition Facts: Calories: 50 | Carbs: 13g | Protein: 0g | Fat: 0g | Fiber: 0g

Ingredients:

- Fruits (kiwi, blueberries, strawberries, orange)
- Half a cup of sugar
- Two teaspoon agar-agar
- Two cups of water

Method:

1. Take a Nagashikan (6 inch×5.1 inch×1.8 inches), and keep it aside.

2. Take a small saucepan and pour two cups of water. Add in two teaspoons of agar-agar. Whisk to combine. Boil.

3. Lower the heat and continue cooking for two minutes. Whisk frequently to ensure that the agar-agar has dissolved completely.

4. Remove from heat after two minutes.

5. Add in one-fourth cup sugar. Whisk until the sugar gets completely dissolved.

6. Pour the liquid in the nagashikan, until it reaches a height of 1/3 inch. This will make sure that the fruits don't touch the bottom.

7. With the help of a toothpick or spoon, move the formed bubbles to the corner and get rid of them.

8. Keep it in the refrigerator for around ten minutes. You can even keep it at room temperature for a slightly longer time.

9. On the other hand, for the jelly, cut the fruits.

10. Make sure that the thickness of the pieces of the fruits is nearly equal.

11. After the bottom layer is nearly set, put the fruit on it.

12. Pour the rest of the mixture on top of it and get rid of the bubbles.

13. Put it inside the refrigerator and keep it there until the jelly is completely set.

14. Run a knife along the sides of the nagashikan to loosen the jelly.

15. Cut the jelly, with the knife, around the sides of the fruits. It will give a pretty look to it.

16. Transfer all the fruit jellies on a plate and serve them chilled.

Warabi Mochi

Total Prep & Cooking Time: 25 minutes

Yields: 4 servings

Nutrition Facts: Calories: 87 | Carbs: 5g | Protein: 0.7g | Fat: 0.5g | Fiber: 0g

Ingredients:

- One and three-fourths of a cup of water
- Half a cup of sugar
- Three-fourth of a cup of Warabiko or Warabi Mochiko

For the toppings:

- Brown sugar syrup (kuromitsu)
- One-fourth cup of kinako

Method:

1. Take a baking sheet and sprinkle some kinako on it.

2. Mix the Warabi Mochiko, water, and sugar in a medium-sized saucepan and heat it over medium heat until it begins to boil.

3. Decrease the heat and stir vigorously using a wooden spatula for about ten minutes so that the mixture thickens and turns translucent.

4. Take the mocha away from the heat and pour it onto the prepared baking sheet. Add some more kinako on the mocha and allow it to cook in the refrigerator for about twenty minutes.

5. Take it out of the refrigerator once it has cooled down and cut in into ¾inch pieces. Add some more kinako on the warabi mocha and serve. You can also add a drizzle of Kuromitsu on top of the mocha if you like.

Notes: *You can store the warabi mocha for one to three days at room temperature. They will get hard and whitish if it's kept in the refrigerator. It also tastes much* *tastier if you keep it in the fridge for twenty to thirty minutes before consuming it.*

Yatsuhashi

Total Prep & Cooking Time: 30 minutes

Yields: Ten pieces

Nutrition Facts: Calories: 532 | Carbs: 64g | Protein: 28g | Fat: 6g | Fiber: 0.8g

Ingredients:

- A quarter cup of rice flour (shiratamako) or mochiko
- A quarter cup and one teaspoon each of
- Water
- Sugar
- One tablespoon of soybean flour (kinako)
- A quarter cup and two teaspoons of rice flour (joshinko)
- One teaspoon of cinnamon powder (mixed with matcha)
- Two teaspoons each of

- Green tea (matcha powder)
- Cinnamon powder
- A two-third cup of bean paste, red (Anko)

Method:

1. In a microwave-safe bowl, add shiratamako and water. Whisk until you no longer find any flour lump. Then add sugar and joshinko. Mix the paste with a spatula to form a slightly thick consistency.

2. Cover the bowl with a plastic wrapper and place it in a microwave oven. The baking time can range from one to three minutes, depending upon the microwave wattage. Take the bowl out after the said time and remix the contents with a wet spatula. Again bake it for one and a half minutes.

3. Remix the contents to form a soft mocha.

4. Cut the dough into thinner pieces of size (0.75-inch x 2.25-inch). Bake them for twenty minutes at a temperature of 150 degrees C. Take it out and serve.

Conclusion

Here we are at the final chapter of this wonderful journey through the taste and delight of Japanese recipes!

Did you have difficulties in the preparation?

Oriental cuisine is not the easiest in the world, but with a little training you can reach very high standards of quality and I am here to teach you how to cook at your best.

Thank you so much for your trust and see you on the next trip!

CPSIA information can be obtained
at www.ICGtesting.com
Printed in the USA
BVHW041755070421
604344BV00012B/1294